YOGA BIBLE

FOR BEGINNERS

50 Best Poses for Beginners, Tips for
Improving Health, Guide on stretching,
Attached Pictures

INNA VOLIA

Contents

Introduction

The practice of yoga is increasingly becoming popular world over with the places that offer yoga practices increasing each day. As much as many people are adopting yoga practice, not many people understand what yoga entirely entails which then limits the benefits that one can experience if they lack sufficient knowledge. **Yoga Bible for Beginners** is a book that has shared in detail what practicing yoga actually entails. The goal of yoga practice is for an individual to get into a state of unity with themselves and with the universal powers.

Yoga practice entails engagement in breathing exercises which helps in enhancing stability in the mind and the body. It also involves engagement in body postures and meditation. All the exercises and techniques are done with the aim of getting the body, mind, and soul into a state of unity with the universal consciousness. Advancement towards that process incorporates the practice of meditation and results into a raised level of awareness as one also gets to experience raised levels of peace and happiness.

While a person is in such a state, they are capable of seeing things in their true nature which then leads to one making the right decisions for their lives. Being in such a state also provides relief from some conditions such as depression, anxiety, and stress alongside other medical conditions. Understanding yoga, the history behind it and all that it entails are therefore vital if one is to realize the benefits associated with the practice. This book has shared in detail what yoga is all about for better understanding.

It has also shared on the history of yoga and the various stages of development that the practice has gone through. The practice of yoga has been embraced by everyone in the society, from the celebrities to the business people, athletes and those from all manner of profession and fields. Yoga has been proven to improve longevity by eliminating various conditions that lead to aging. It also eliminates conditions such as stress, anxiety and such like. Practicing yoga puts one into an enhanced state of awareness, happiness, and peace.

As a beginner, avoid any form of high goals and competition as such may hinder you from realizing the great benefits. Remember that the time one takes to master a given posture or meditation technique may not be the same for all. That's why it's vital that you just ensure that you practice yoga regularly even if you only spend five minutes a day. Before you know it, the benefits that may seem to be subtle at the beginning can turn into great and life-changing ones if the practice is sustained. Practicing yoga also causes one to be watchful over their body, it the results in one becoming more keen on how their actions have contributed to the present states of their bodies.

A person who is overweight will be keen on the type of foods they eat and such conscious way of living then results into sustained healthy life. Take your time to read the book all through and try out some of the shared yoga postures. Remember to practice regularly for better-improved life and sustained results.

Chapter 1

What is Yoga

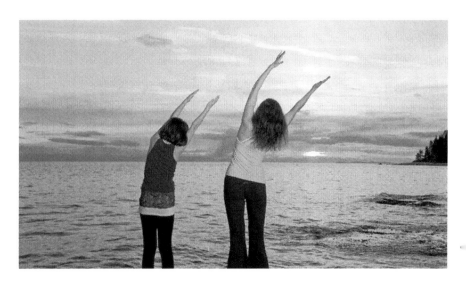

So many things come and go with trends that keep changing time after time but the practice of yoga has been around for the past 15,000 years. Yoga has survived all the distortion and transmission challenges and still stands out as one of the oldest practices that are embraced world over. The survival of yoga has been sustained mainly because it's not a practice that's forced on anyone. It's a process of well being that one gets to voluntarily embrace if they intend to realize the numerous benefits associated with the practice. Yoga and meditation have become some of the popular ways that those who seek wellbeing tend to adopt.

Yoga is a combination of physical, spiritual and mental practices that are done with the aim of achieving unity of the mind, body, and spirit with the universal force. The word yoga comes from a Sanskrit word yuj which means union, to bind or yoke. The main goal of engaging in yoga practice is to bring the mind into experiencing a deeper state of connection which then enables one to realize deeper states of consciousness. As a beginner, there are some crucial aspects of yoga that you should understand clearly if your yoga practice is to yield great results. The pressures of life have pushed people into a life of internal turmoil leading to high levels and anxiety; many people practicing yoga have been influenced into the practice mostly because of yoga's ability to provide relief from such conditions.

Understanding Yoga Practice

The journey of practicing yoga stems from developing a strong desire to live a peaceful and harmonious life. As much as a beginner may not be well aware of that deeper yearning; the desire will get much stronger when they begin to experience that connection between the breath with the body, mind, and spirit. Yoga can, therefore, be described as a state of harmony that people get to lose due to the busy and fast-paced nature of the world. The evolution of yoga into very powerful spiritual discipline starts with a lot of humility and should be practiced in such a subtle and gentle way and not in a forceful way of building muscles as expressed in other forms of exercises. Remember that may create resistance and that's what you're working to eliminate.

There are different factors that drive people into practicing yoga. Some get involved in the practice for various benefits such as health benefits, weight loss, and flexibility while others enjoy being in an attractive body that's vibrant and fit. There are also those who feel overwhelmed with chaos of the outside world and often turn to yoga as a way of practicing mindfulness and being in the moment. Yoga is not just about the postures, engaging in yoga postures is just a part of the exercise.

Focusing on postures alone may not provide all the life-improving benefits that one can get from the practice. Practicing yoga as a spiritual path leads in a way of happiness, contentment, and awareness.

A beginner's mind just like a child's heart is willing to trust the process, to love and to learn something, which then causes a beginner to attain higher levels of awareness in a much easier way. For a beginner to enjoy all the benefits that come with yoga, they should not just practice it as a way of engaging in physical exercise but as a spiritual path that leads to enhanced states of awareness. When you start out with yoga practice as a beginner, avoid setting goals that are way to high instead try to embrace yoga practice as a way of life geared towards attaining unity and harmony with the inner self and the spiritual forces. Setting higher expectations may live you so much focused on the end results and that can deprive you of experiencing the joy and fun of being in the moment.

The practice of yoga entails engagement in physical exercises in the form of postures. As much as some postures look easy and you may start to practice immediately without the help of a trainer, there are postures that can only be mastered after several months of practice such as the one's involving full back bend and other complex poses. As a beginner, don't be in a hurry to master the complex poses, take your time as you engage in the practice and allow your body to grow gradually into the postures. Forcing yourself to be perfect in the complex poses before the body gets well aligned may only lead pain and injuries. Yoga practice has the potential of teaching one endurance, patience and other values that make life to be fun and exciting.

Instead of spending your days in worry, stress and anxiety, practicing yoga teach one breathing techniques that enables one to see things with clarity and in their true nature. Once you are able to see things clearly then you will realize that you don't have to worry about things that are yet to come or of those things of the past. Your focus will then be in the present moment where you dedicate yourself to being in the moment. When practicing yoga, it's good to know that your body has a memory structure that if you are willing to monitor and understand then you will realize how your actions have contributed to the state your body is in.

Yoga practice provides a way of opening up hat memory structure so that you are able to restructure your life in a way that provides you with ultimate possibility in life. It's such a subtle and scientific process that if well practiced, has the potential of transforming one's life to greater levels of peace, joy, and awareness.

Chapter 2

History of Yoga

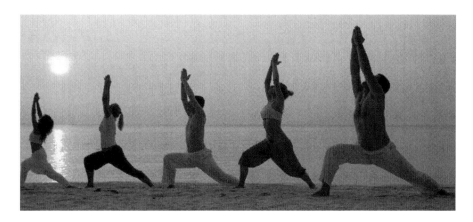

The oral translation of the sacred texts and the secretive nature of yoga teachings have led in some way to the misunderstanding of what the practice entailed. The early yoga writings were transcribed on palm leaves which were very fragile and got damaged easily or even got lost. The original development of yoga goes back to over 5000 years ago. The rich history can, therefore, be divided into main periods such as innovation, development, and practice. The practice of yoga was developed over 5000 years ago by the Indus-Sarasvati in Northern India.

The mention of the word yoga was found in the sacred texts, Rig Veda. These were a collection of texts that contained songs, mantras, and rituals which were used by the Vedic priests, Brahmans. Yoga then got refined slowly and was developed by the priests and the mystic seers who then documented the beliefs and practice of yoga into Upanishads, a huge collection that consisted of over 200 scriptures. One of the most renowned recordings of yogic scriptures is found in the Bhagavad-Gita which was composed around the period 500 B.C.E. The Upanishads embraced the idea of ritualistic sacrifice from the Vedas which they managed to internalize as they taught about the sacrifice of the ego through action or karma yoga, self-knowledge, and wisdom, jnana yoga.

How yoga practice evolved

During the pre-classical stage, the practice of yoga was a mixture of various ideas, techniques, and beliefs and often they contradicted each other. This period is defined by Patanjali's yoga sutras that presented yoga in a systematic way. It was written around the second century and it entails the path of Raja yoga which was organized by Patanjali into the eight-limbed path. Raja yoga expresses steps and stages that should be taken towards the attainment of enlightenment. Patanjali is considered by many as the father of yoga and the yoga sutras still have a strong influence on most styles of the modern yoga.

After a few centuries, yoga masters came up with a set of practices that were designed to help in rejuvenating the body and prolonging life. They did away with the ancient Vedas teachings and focused on the physical body as the ideal way to achieve enlightenment. They developed a practice known as Tantra yoga which entailed radical techniques that were aimed at cleansing the mind and body with the aim of breaking the knots that tends to bind people to their physical existence. This exploration of physical and spiritual connections and other body-centered practices then led to the creation of the present type of Hatha yoga which is commonly practiced in the West.

During the 18th and 19th Centuries, yoga masters started traveling to the West where they attracted the attention of numerous followers. In 1893 during a session in the Parliament of Religions which took place in Chicago, Swami Vivekananda excited the crowd through his lectures on yoga practice and about the universal nature of the world religions. Hatha yoga grew in popularity in India in the 1920s to 30s and yoga student were produced that would continue with the practice and popularity of Hatha yoga. Many yoga teachers became pioneers of the practice and even opened yoga studios in the West. Yoga practice has greatly grown into popularity world over with many people embracing the different aspects of the practice.

Yoga practice has become a common path for those looking for ways to attain overall wellbeing. There are various facets of yoga such as breathing techniques, the moral principles and the poses that many people find to be appealing and beneficial. Most of the people world over from celebrities, athletes, business people, and all others find the process of yoga practice to be subtle and easy to adopt and that's something that has led to its popularity. The practice of yoga is geared towards connection. It entails connection with the inner self, who we truly are and connection with the planet and the universe at large.

Chapter 3

How Yoga improves Life and Health

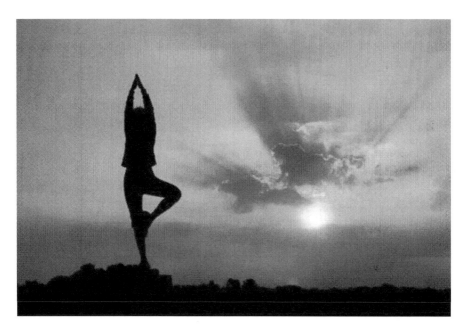

Yoga is a practice that has been misunderstood by many people with some seeing it as part of a religion but yoga practice offers more than one can only get to know of by embracing the practice. Yoga practice is not just about postures and exercises but a complete guide to living a more fulfilled, healthy and productive life. Practicing yoga is not only beneficial to the body but equally to the mind, the spirit and the soul as well. There are numerous ways through which yoga practice have been proven to be beneficial. The benefits associated with yoga practice have been documented through the years and they range from relief from stress and depression, raised energy and vitality levels, increased feelings of happiness and overall well being amongst others.

As a beginner starting out, it's important that you view yoga as a way of cultivating unity between your mind, body, soul, and spirit and aligning yourself with the universal forces. You will then be able to view every technique in the process as a way of helping you advance towards attaining that goal of connection. Yoga practice can also be embraced as a way of improving life and overall wellness of the body, however, the practice should not be only limited to attaining the desired benefits. It's something that should be practiced regularly even after the desired goal is realized whether its weight loss, good health, and such life. There are numerous ways through which yoga helps to improve life and below are some of them.

Relief from some mental illnesses
As much as more research is still being undertaken in this area, there are some great finding suggesting that practicing yoga can immensely help with addressing some medical conditions such as schizophrenia, ADHD, depression and such like. Engaging in yoga practice can give one relief from the use of antidepressants that also come with side effects if used for a longer period of time. Cultivating a state of mindfulness with breathing exercises helps with enabling the mind to be still and while in that state, chemicals that enhance states of happiness gets release which then heightens relief from such condition. A person experiencing such mental illnesses should, therefore, ensure they engage in all the areas of practicing yoga.

They can focus on poses to help with breath practice and then advance to mindfulness and meditation which will, in turn, lead to such desired state. Incorporating meditation which is also part of yoga practice enables one to rise to levels of awareness where the body, mind, and spirit get to operate in unity and that helps in cultivating that element of calmness and peace of mind. Practicing yoga also improves the help of the brain. Through a practice of mindfulness meditation, the grey matter and volume of the brain get to increase especially for those who have developed meditation as a daily practice.

Engaging in mantra meditation can also help in enhancing cognitive health. Taking a few minutes each day in meditation helps in increasing activity in the brain areas that are responsible for memory and that can help with relief from diseases such as dementia and Alzheimer.

Enhances flexibility and bone health

Practicing yoga poses helps in enhancing mobility and body balance and muscle strength. As one engages in yoga practice, they get to exercise muscles that would otherwise be dormant and fragile. Having strong muscles helps with prevention of diseases such as arthritis and back pain. It also helps with prevention of unnecessary falls especially with the elderly. It then leads to body vitality and flexibility which causes one to handle some tasks efficiently that would have otherwise been a challenge. Engaging in yoga exercises also enables one to stretch every part of the body which then results in the overall health of the body. All round wellness is not just about being physically fit, its being in a state of energetic flow and vitality.

When one is full of life energy and vitality, they are capable of thinking clearly and executing tasks in a way that's fulfilling. They get to put that level of focus and energy into all that they engage in. Exercising also helps in body alignment which then leads to improved body posture. Engaging in weight-bearing exercises helps in strengthening bones and also helps with warding off conditions such as osteoporosis. Many of the yoga postures require people get to carry their own weight with others helping with the strengthening of the arms. Practicing yoga helps with lowering the levels of cortisol, a hormone that responsible for causing stress.

Weight reduction

Many people get into practices like addiction to junk foods and other unhealthy eating habits that lead to weight gain and this happens mostly due to stress and anxiety. Since engaging in yoga practice enables one to overcome stress and anxiety, one is ten able to think clearly and be able to make the right choices that help in improving their overall wellbeing. By practicing yoga, one also engages in exercises that impact every part of the body including inner organs such as the heart and kidney muscles. The regular practice of yoga enables one to attain their desired body weight that they can easily maintain as they get to be more aware of their body and how they should relate to it.

A person that's more aware of their body will avoid consuming food that makes them feel more sluggish and lethargic. They will instead go for foods that are healthy and helps in improving overall body vitality.

Increases blood flow

Practicing yoga helps in increasing the flow of blood through the body. Engaging in relaxation exercises helps with improved circulation all through the body. Yoga practice also helps in improving the flow of oxygen to the body cells. Postures such as headstand or shoulder stand encourage the flow of blood from the pelvis area and the legs to flow back to the heart. Yoga practice helps with boosting levels of red blood cells and hemoglobin which carries oxygen to the body tissues. It thins the blood and reduces the level of blood clotting and also helps in reducing cases of strokes and heart attack.

Improves heart rate

Getting your heart to regular aerobic range helps in lowering the rates of heart attack and also relieves anxiety and depression. Yoga exercise also helps in improving cardiovascular conditioning. Various studies have proven that yoga practice helps in lowering the resting heart rate while also increasing the level of endurance and that improves maximum uptake of oxygen, especially during exercise times. Those who have engaged in breathing exercises can do many exercises with less oxygen intake which is great.

Drops of blood pressure

Practicing yoga is quite beneficial to those with high blood pressure condition. Engaging in simple yoga postures like the corpse pose can greatly impact and lower the blood pressure. Practicing yoga also helps in regulating the adrenal glands. Engaging in breathing exercises and meditation helps in lowering the levels of cortisol and that result into improved system. High levels of cortisol may cause changes in the brain that can have long-term impact.

Practicing yoga also stimulates the organs such as the kidneys and the liver leading to activation of the natural detoxification process. Any twist in body posture increases enhances the cleansing process.

Improves awareness and concentration

Practicing meditation and breathing techniques ushers one into a level of awareness and while in such a state they get to experience ultimate peace with enhanced levels of awareness. Practicing mindfulness and living in the moment is one of the benefits associated with yoga and leads one into experiencing feelings of joy, peace, and happiness. Practicing focus enhances one's level of concentration and one's one to be free from a wondering mind. This is a great benefit as one is able to achieve a lot within a given time if wondering and restlessness are controlled.

Yoga also enables one to test their body limits and the extent one can go. By engaging in the yoga postures one can know the extent of exercises that their bodies can be capable of. Seeing yourself advance from basic postures to intermediary and the advanced ones also help in boosting one's level of confidence and self-belief. Yoga awakens a strong feeling from within that causes one to be steadfast in their practice that leads to being in sync with self. The changes that take place when one is practicing yoga may be quite subtle and small but when the practice is carried out consistently, the cumulative benefits of the benefits then begins to feature significantly and before you know it, you realize that you're less anxious, less stressed and with sustained levels of happiness.

Promotes longevity

Yoga practice involves techniques and exercises that have the potential of enhancing longevity. A number of studies undertaken about the practice have revealed that yoga practice can address some age-related health problems effectively. Some of the ways through which yoga can be used to increase longevity include;

Yoga can help with addressing age-related respiratory ailments. A study of human kinetics revealed that engaging in a 12-week yoga practice helped with influencing the respiratory functioning in the elderly women. Yoga practice also helps in improving memory capacity and efficiency. It also addresses cases related to cognitive decline. Yoga also helps in slowing oxidation process which is attributed to speeding the aging process. The stretching, inhaling and exhaling that takes place during the breathing process promotes oxygenation and dilation to the body tissues and thus increases longevity. Yoga does that but enhancing the use of oxygen throughout the entire body which then leads to the release of free radicals which contributes to the gradual corrosion of the body.

Yoga slows the breath rate which then makes one a slow and deep breather. It then reduces oxidation rate which then leads to a longer lifespan. Intake of deep breaths also helps with activation of the parasympathetic nervous system which enables one to stay calm and relaxed. Practicing yoga generally causes to live a peaceful long life.

Tips to Guide Yoga Practice

Before you start off with yoga practice as a beginner, there are some things that you should put in place to ensure that your practice session flows well;

- Before doing yoga, you should ensure that you take food two hours earlier to the practice time. This is to help with your digestive system so that you don't get interrupted during the process of practice. Remember excessive intake of spicy food is also not recommended during yoga practice.

- Take time for some warm ups before the practice as it helps in preparing the muscles and the nerves. In case you are practicing in a studio that has others as well, remember to avoid causing any of disturbances especially to those who are in a concentrated and focused mode.

- As much as yoga entails engaging in exercises, the desired results can only be realized with internal focus. Every exercise should, therefore, be carried out with internal focus. When your focus is outward on the techniques and how you are working it out, you may find yourself having difficulty during the practice sessions.

- When going to practice, ensure that you wear comfortable clothing. As you will be able to see in the next chapters, most of the postures are done in a spacious environment with comfortable clothing.

- Avoid being too strict with yourself remember you're not competing against anyone so let your focus be more inward on your breathing and feelings and not on perfect pose or exercise.

Chapter 4

Practice 50 poses for beginners

1. Easy Pose

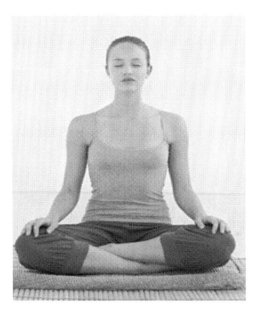

Steps

- Sit on the floor with your legs stretched before you and your back straight

- Cross your legs as demonstrated in the pose with the knees broadened until your legs and thighs form into a triangle.

- Keep some space between your feet and your pelvis with your back raised as you focus your gaze ahead.

- Inhale and exhale five deep breaths as you stay in the position.

Benefits

- Stretches the legs and arms while also lengthening the spine

- Opens up the hips and provides relief from menstrual pains.

- Lowers anxiety and calms the mind

- Enhances peace and serenity

2. Triangle Pose

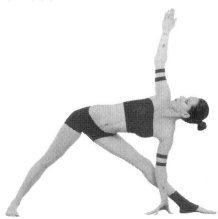

Steps

- Stand straight as you and keep both your feet apart.

- Turn the right leg to about 90 degrees a shown in the pose then breathe in.

- Bend the left side of your body while you exhale with your right hand facing upwards and the left hand touching your left toe.

- Take five deep breaths as you stay in the pose for about a minute then changes to the other side.

Benefits

- Improves flexibility and alignment of both the spine and the shoulders

- Provides relief from body stiffness and areas around the neck area and back.

- Stretches and strengthens the body and also improves circulation of blood circulation while also stimulating the functioning of the kidneys.

3. Four limbed staff

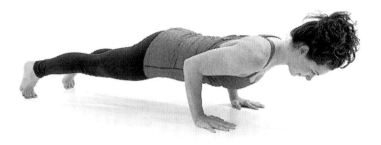

Steps

- Begin with all four then step your feet back like in a push-up position as shown in the pose above.

- Spread your fingers apart wide as you press your palms and arms straight.

- Tuck your tail bone so that torso, hips, and the legs stay in a straight line.

- Press your head and shoulders forward with your toss tucked inside as you press your heels back.

- Take five deep breaths as you stay in the position then repeat a few times and release.

Benefits

- Strengthens and stretches the abdomen, arms, and the wrists. The pose is also suitable for practice when practicing the arm balancing poses that could be challenging.

- Lengthens the spine and also strengthens the low back muscles and the spine

4. Warrior pose

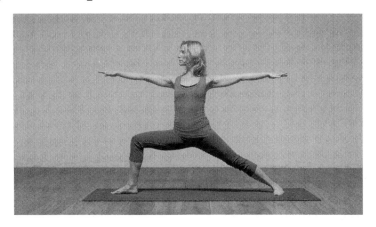

Steps

- Begin in a standing position with your legs straight apart.

- Inhale deeply as you raise both your hands up then turn your head towards the right.

- Exhale while you turn the right foot to about 90 degrees towards the right.

- Bend your knees with both your hands stretched and parallel to the mat then hold on to the position as you take seven deep breaths.

- Repeat with your left leg while you also turn your head towards the left.

Benefits

- Increases stamina and body flexibility

- Strengthens and stretches the legs, the lower back, and the arms while also toning the lower body.

- Strengthens the abdominal organs and also improves blood circulation all the entire body.

- Provides relief from stress and body pains while also improving concentration.

5. Tree Pose

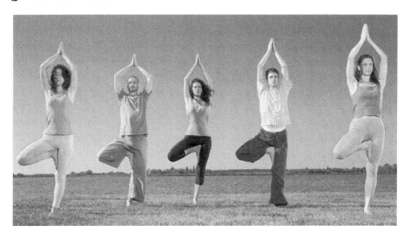

Steps

- Stand straight as your arms rest by your side then find balance as you place the sole of your right foot on the left thigh and it should be slightly above your knee.

- Once you have attained balance, raise both hands up and bring them into prayer position.

- Stay in the position as you take five deep breaths then change to the other leg.

Benefits

- Helps in improving balance for the body while also strengthening the muscles and the thighs, calves, ankles, legs and the spine.

6. Child Pose

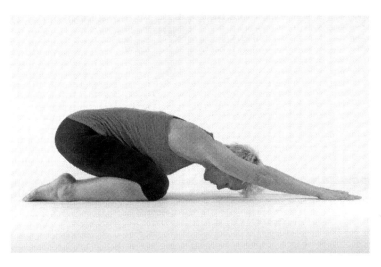

Steps

- Begin in a kneeling position then stretch your hands forward with your palms on the mat as you lean on your thighs

- Let your thighs stay as shown in the above pose then bring your chest closer to the knees as you stretch your hands forward.

- Stay in the position as you take five deep breaths then stay in then repeat for about three minutes. Breathe gently as you hold on the posture for about 3 minutes

- Come back to the starting position then repeat the cycle 6 times or more.

Benefits

- Cures back pains while also releasing tension, stress, and fatigue.

- Stretches the thighs, hips, and ankles while also relaxing front body muscles

7. Bridge Posture

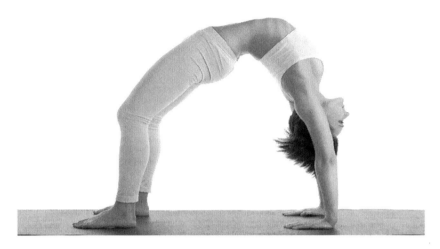

Steps

- Lie on your back then lift the upper and lower body parts of the body as shown in the pose.

- Push your spine in as your head relaxes between your arms

- Stay in the position as you take five deep breaths

- Repeat the cycle 5 times as you take deep breaths in between

Benefits

- Opens up the hip joints and strengthens the heart and chest muscles.

- Strengthens the chest and also strengthens the spinal muscles.

- Reduces stress and increases blood flow to the upper parts of the body

8. Quarter Dog

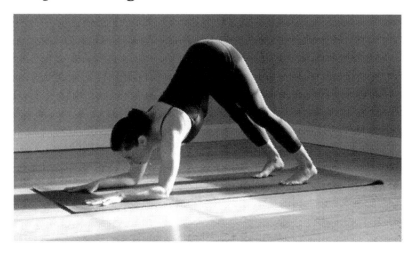

Steps

- Begin by bending your hands and knees as you rest your wrists underneath the shoulders with your knees beneath the hips.

- Take a deep breath as you place your toes beneath your knees then exhale as you lift the hips.

- Your posture should create a straight line between the elbows and your middle fingers.

- Straighten the fingers as you lower your arms and straighten the legs then lower your heels.

- Relax your head between your arms as you focus your gaze towards your belly.

- Hold on to the position as you take five deep breaths.

Benefits

- Stretches and strengthens the lower back, hamstrings, and the calves.

- Transfers weight from the hands and wrists.

9. Breathing Pose

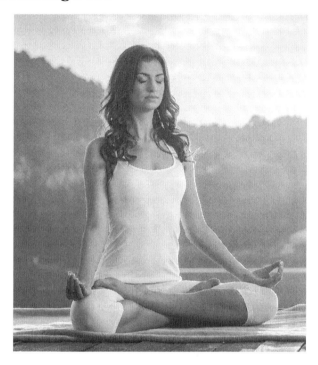

Steps

- Sit with you back straight on the mat and your head focused and raised

- Cross your legs in lotus position as you rest your hands on your ankles.

- Stay in the pose as you inhale a deep breath through your nose then exhale through the mouth as you make a whoosh noise.

Benefits

- Improves the glow and beauty of the skin and also enhances the working of the lungs.

- Strengthens the heart muscles while also normalizes the heart rate.

10.   Corpse pose

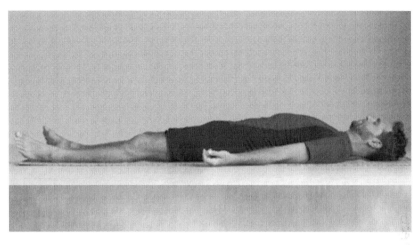

Steps

- Lie down flat on the mat and close your eyes

- Let your mind be free of all negative thoughts while you relax completely

- Lie straight with your leg apart as you take deep long breaths

- Exhale slowly then stay in the position as you repeat the process about 5 times.

Benefits

- Relaxes the mind and the body while also enabling one to release stress the stress they are carrying

- Improves flexibility, balance, and strengthens the entire body

- Creates a peaceful association with death.

11. Bow Pose

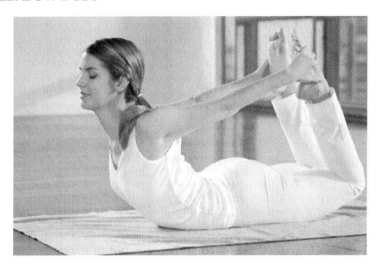

Steps

- Begin by lying on your stomach with the hands right by your side

- Bend your knees slightly then bring the heels closer to your buttocks.

- Stretch the hands to hold your ankles as you slightly pull them together while your torso rises.

- Your body should take the shape of a bow.

- Stay in the position as you take five deep breaths then relax and repeat several times.

Benefits

- Strengthens and stretches the back muscles, the arms, legs, and the abdomen.

- Tones the muscles and also cultivates a healthy and supple spine.

- Improves the body posture and increases stability.

12. Headstand Pose

Steps

- Place your head on the mat I a haling position with your arms around the head

- Interlock your arms behind the head as your elbows stay on the mat.

- Take deep breaths as you stretch your body as shown in the pose. You can begin by lifting one leg then establish balance as you raise the other leg.

- As a beginner is advisable that you practice this pose with the help of a guide or teacher.

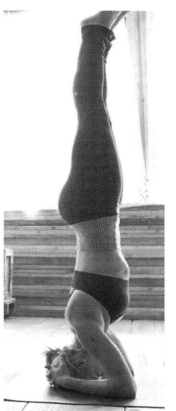

Benefits

- Enhances focus and relieves stress

- Improves blood flow to the upper parts of the body including the head and the eyes.

- Strengthens the shoulders and the arms

13. The wind Relieving Pose

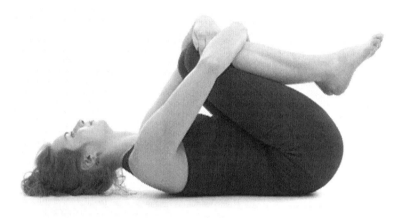

Steps

- Lie on your back with your knees drawn closer to the chest then wrap your arms around the knees

- Wrap your arms around your knees with your legs held closer together.

- Raise your head upwards as you stay in the position then take five deep breaths.

Benefits

- Stretches the leg muscles and speeds up recovery from injury

- Releases tension on the thighs, lower back, and hips

- Relieves indigestion, bloating, acidity and constipation

14. Extended Boat Pose

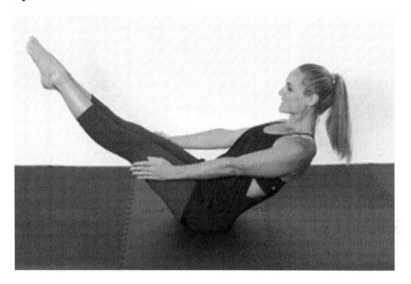

Steps

- Sit on your hips with your legs stretched ahead of you then place your hands on the hips as you gain balance.

- Raise your legs above the mat as you push the stomach inwards then stretch both of your arms beside your thigh.

- Raise your legs to a V shape as in the pose above or to about 45 degrees

- Stay in the position as you take five breaths.

Benefits

- Builds your core strength and also enhances endurance.

- Relieves gas and bloating while also strengthening the abdominal muscles.

- Strengthens and strengthens the spine

15. Happy Baby Pose

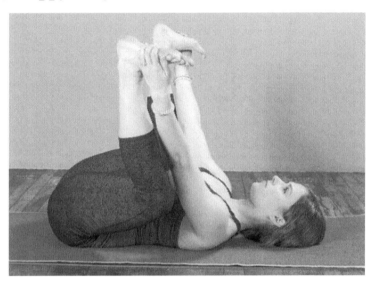

Steps

- Lie on a mat then pull your knees closer to the chest as shown in the pose

- Place your hands on your feet as you open your knees to be wider than your torso.

- Use your hand to press your feet inwards then pull down your feet so as to create some resistance.

- Stay in the position as you take five deep breaths then you can practice the pose for about 3 minutes

Benefits

- Opens up the hips and tones he inner thighs and the groin areas
- Stretches the hamstrings and also relieves the lower back pain
- Soothes and stretches the spine and the abdominal muscles
- Relieves fatigue and stress

16. Butterfly pose

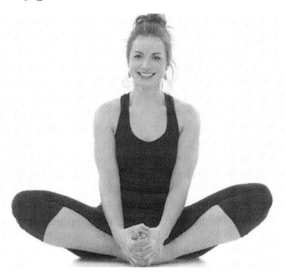

Steps

- Begin in a sitting position with your spine straight and your knees bent as you pull your feet closer to yourself as possible.

- Try and touch the soles of your feet as you hold with hands as shown in the pose.

- Flap like a butterfly as you bring your thighs up and down at a slow pace for about 2 minutes

Benefits

- Improves the functioning of abdominal organs including the prostate glands, kidneys, and the bladder.

17. Reclining Hero Pose

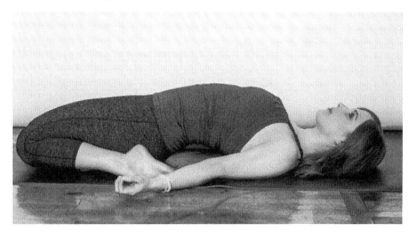

Steps

- Begin by kneeling on the mat with the thighs perpendicular to the floor and the upper part of your feet facing down.

- Slide your feet slightly apart so that they are wider than the hips then press your feet down on the mat.

- Sit down slowly between your feet with your hands turned upwards beside your feet

- Lean backward then lower your torso to the mat

- Stay in the position as you take five or more deep breaths then release.

Benefits

- Strengthens and relaxes the legs and provides relief from back pains

- Improves digestion and relaxes the abdominal muscles

- Provides relief from body pains

18. King dancer pose

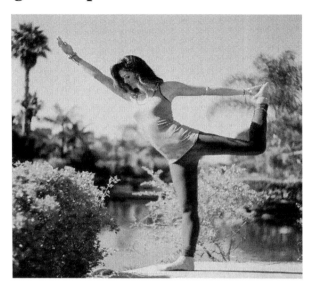

Steps

- Stand tall as you distribute the body to the feet as per the pose

- Let your weight shift to the right foot then bend your left knee while you lift your left feet up above the floor.

- Hold your left foot using the left hand as your thumb rests on the sole of your foot.

- Lift your right arm straight upwards as you also squeeze your left foot

- Stay in that position as you take 10 breaths then change to the other foot.

Benefits

- Strengthens the legs and improves overall body balance.

- Improves core body strength and also stretches muscles

- Enhances focus and concentration

19.Cobra pose

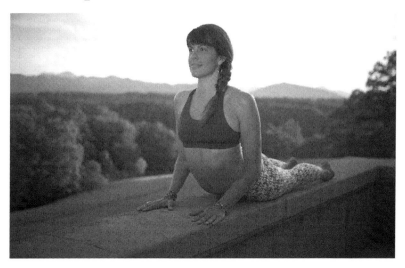

Steps

- Lie down on your belly as you take a deep breath then raise the upper part of your body and chest as shown in the pose.

- Your head and shoulders should be raises straight with your pals resting on the floor

- Stay in that position as you exhale as you raise the upper part of the body off the ground.

- Take five deep breaths while in the position then repeat the posture five times.

Benefits

- Strengthens the abdominal muscles and relieves constipation, indigestion, and acidity.

- Reduces belly fat and also improves blood circulation

- Strengthens shoulder muscles and upper body parts

20. **Twisted Seated Pose**

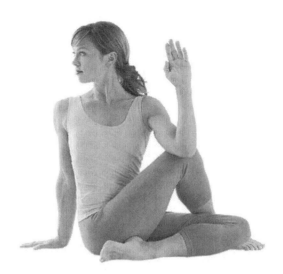

Steps

- Sit on the floor with your legs crossed as in the pose and your hands stretched to the sides.

- Take deep breaths as you shift the left hand to the right thigh then twist your torso.

- Breathe out as you twist the body and hold on that position for about thirty seconds then repeat on the left side.

Benefits

- Strengthens the spine and also improves the overall well being

- Improves the functioning of the digestive system

- Improves the normal spinal rotation

- Relieves stress

21.Sage Pose

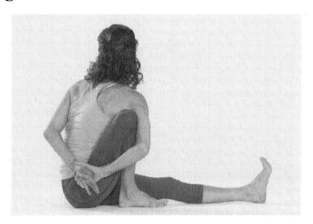

Steps

- Begin with sitting on the floor and then stretch your legs forward. Bend the right knee as your toes remain flat on the ground and your feet drawn closer to the pelvis.

- Bring the left knee close to your chest with the toes facing upwards.

- Let your spine stay straight as you stretch your shoulder and arms on both sides.

- Take a deep breath while you twist the upper body from your waist towards the left slowly.

- Wrap the arms while you slowly bend your knees while also ensuring that they remain straight.

- Inhale deep breaths as you also let your head and shoulder face towards the opposite direction.

- Hold onto the position as you breathe normally then change to the other side.

Benefits

- Stimulates the brain and also enables the body to
- Stretches the shoulders and the spine
- Provides relief from backache and other body pain.

22.   **Warrior Lunge Twist**

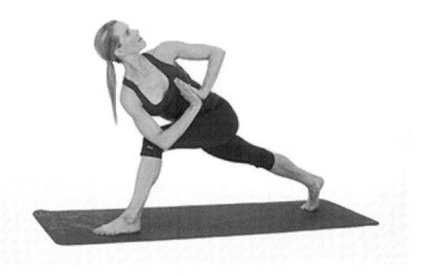

Steps

- Begin by bringing your hands into a prayer pose then stretch forward with the left leg bent to about 90 degrees.

- Keep your back straight as you brace the abs tightly closer to your spine.

- Twist the upper part of your body towards the left as you also keep your spine straight then lean over on your left leg.

- Press your right elbow outside of the left leg then turn your head as if looking upwards over to the left shoulder.

- Stay in the position as you take 10 deep breaths and while in the position then repeat with the other side

Benefits

- Stretches and strengthens parts of the body that are the hard to tone

- Improves body stability and flexibility while also improving blood   flow

23.   Warrior III

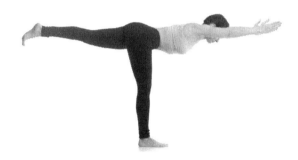

Steps

- Begin by standing on both your feet then shift your weight to your right foot as you straighten your back to be parallel with the ground just as sown in the pose

- Flex your left foot while you point the toes down.

- Stretch your arms straight ahead of you so that your body is straight right from the fingertips down to the back and heel.

- Stay in the position for a few seconds as you take five deep and long breaths then slowly return to a standing position then repeat on the other side.

Benefits

- Strengthens and stretches the legs and also opens up the hips

- Improves blood circulation and also increases respiration

- Energizes the entire body

- Provides healing from injuries.

24.   Lotus Hip Lift

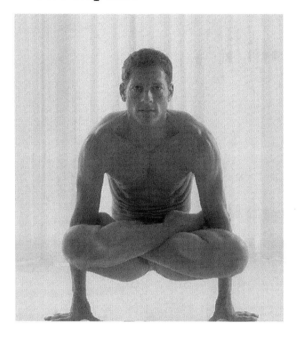

Steps

- Sit on the floor with your crossed legs crossed then press your palms on the hips.

- Your fingertips should be pressed on the floor as you brace your abs as shown in the pose and press your arms down.

- Lift your hips off the mat as you transfer weight to the hands then hold in the position as you take three breaths

- Lower then release and repeat a few times.

Benefits

- Straightens and strengthens the spine while also enhancing awareness and attentiveness

- Calms the brain and provides relief from stress

25. Wide legged Forward Bend

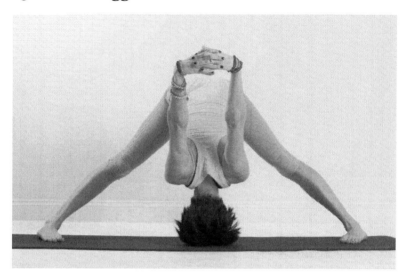

Steps

- Stand on your feet with your legs apart and your heels facing outwards.

- Stand tall while you interlace your hands behind as you press the palms together.

- Take deep long breaths as you fold your waist while you lower and stretch your hand.

- Stretch your back straight then stay in the position as you take 5 deep breaths.

- Repeat the pose five times then release

Benefits

- Opens up tight hamstrings

- Improves blood circulation throughout the body.

- Enhances digestion and stretches the abdominal muscles

26.   Half Moon

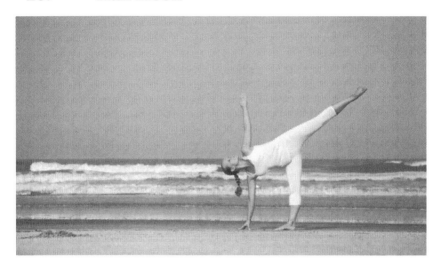

Steps

- Start in the downward facing dog position as you step forward with your right foot then rise into warrior 1 position.

- Open your chest, your arms, and hips as you place your hand on the left hip while you also stretch the arm straight out.

- Shift the body weight into your right foot then lift your left foot

- Place the right palm right on the ground beneath the shoulder as you bend the right knee.

- Stretch your left arm up straight then raise your head as you look towards the raised arm.

- Stay in the position as you take five breaths then try the half moon pose on your left side.

Benefits

- Strengthens and stretches the body and reduces the back fat

- Strengthens the hamstring, groins, and the calves.

27. Extended wide squat

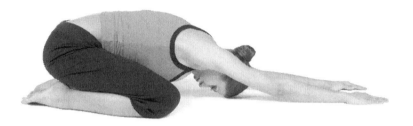

Steps

- Begin in a squatting position as you let your legs slightly apart. Stretch your hands on the floor as you lean forward while also pressing your belly on your thighs towards the floor.

- Relax your head between your hands as you lower it on the mat.

Benefits

- Stretches and relaxes the spine and the hips.

- Calms the head and relaxes the arms.

- Strengthens the abdominal areas.

28.   Plough Pose

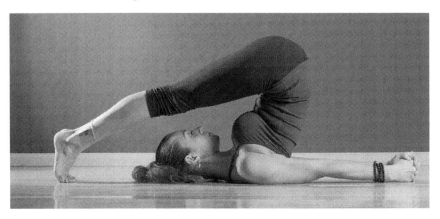

Steps

- Begin by lying on the mat on your back with your arms placed by your side. Lift up your feet until your angle forms between the upper and lower torso.

- Lift your hips off the mat slowly as you also use the hands for balance.

- Lift your legs up and allow them to touch the mat right beyond your head. It should be similar to the pose above. Your body should look more like an arch.

- Stay in the position as you take fie deep breaths then release and repeat three times.

Blessings

- Stretches the muscles and stimulates the internal organs

- Strengthens and stretches the shoulders, thyroid, and the hamstrings.

- Improves spines flexibility.

29.   Wheel Pose

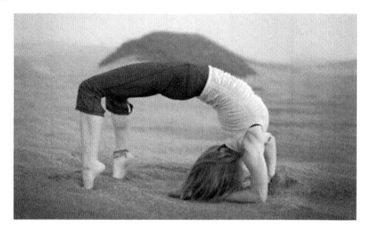

Steps

- Begin by lying on your back as you bend the knees then place your feet on the ground. Bend your elbows as you place your palms on the ground in the above pose above.

- Take a deep breath as you press your palms and lift your head off the ground then exhale.

- Take a deep breath while in the pose then try to walk with your hands with your feet closer together.

- Stay in the position for five deep breaths then lower your body down slowly down.

- Repeat the pose three times then relax.

Benefits

- Increases flexibility and strengthens the spine and shoulders.

- Strengthens the upper body as you also stretch the abs and the quads which make it ideal for runners.

30. Camel pose

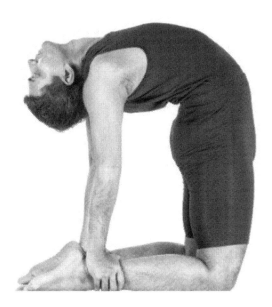

Steps

- Begin by kneeling down on the mat then bend your back until your palms touch your feet.

- Lower your shoulders and head as you raise your chest upwards as in the pose.

- Hold onto the pose as you take deep seven breaths.

Benefits

- Stretches and strengthens the deep hip flexors and also opens up the hips

- Stretches and strengthens the spine and the shoulder back

- Opens up the chest and also improves respiration

- Provides relief to the lower back pain.

31. Sliding Table

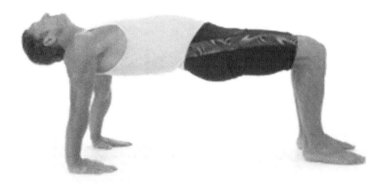

Steps

- Begin by sitting on the mat then bend your knees with your feet flat on the mat and your hip wide.

- Place your hands on your hips and your fingertips facing towards your body slightly.

- Raise your hips so as to appear in a table top position just as in the pose.

- Stretch your legs as you push your hips back as you raise the pelvis behind the hips.

- Stay in the position as you hold five deep breaths.

Benefits

- Stretches and strengthen the spine, back, shoulder, chest and the spine

- Strengthens and stretches the muscles around the spine.

32.   **Stacked side Plank**

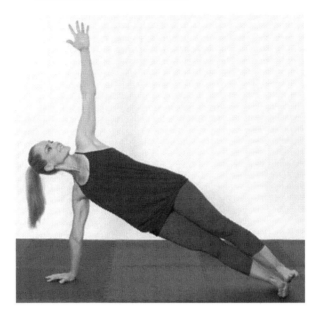

Steps

- Begin by lying on the right side then straighten your knees.

- Place your right hand beneath the shoulder then raise your hips off the mat as your body takes the shape of a straight line right from your ankles up to the shoulders.

- Stretch your left arm upwards towards the ceiling as you take a deep breath

- Hold on to the position for five deep breaths or for about 60 seconds. You can then lower and repeat the posture with the other side.

Benefits

- Strengthens and stretches the entire body including the abdominal area.

- Tones the body and relaxes the feet muscles.

33.   Side Fierce

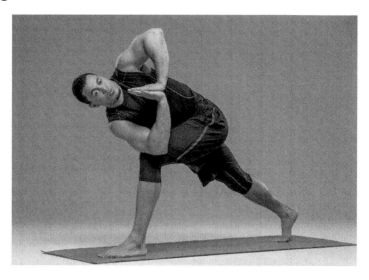

Steps

- Begin in a standing position as you place both your feet close on the floor

- Bend your knees then squat into the fierce pose as you rotate your torso then cross your right elbow outside of the right thigh.

- Press your arms closer as you lift your torso then pull your right hip back so that your knees line in order to keep the weight back on the heels.

- Take five deep breaths as you hold the position then turn your gaze over to the left shoulder.

Benefits

- Strengthens your shoulders, arms, and the wrists

- Strengthens and stretches the legs and also improves balance

- Improves focus and concentration

34.   Arching three legged dog

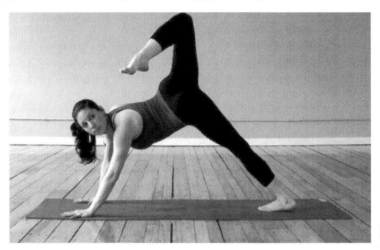

Steps

- Begin in the side fierce pose then take the posture of a downward facing dog.

- Place both of your feet together while you leave the left heel on the mat then raise your right leg upwards as you bend the knee.

- Squeeze your right heel towards the hips then lift your knee high.

- Lift up your head as you turn and look over to your shoulder and the arching spine.

- Stay in the position as you take five deep breaths while also keeping the belly still and breathe through your chest.

Benefits

- Stretches and strengthens your entire body

- Rejuvenates the brain

35.   Open side fierce

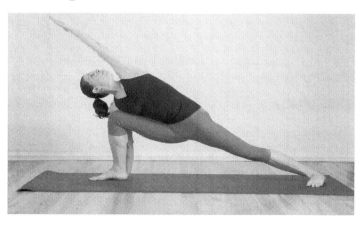

Steps

- Start in a standing position with both of your feet together then bend the knees and squat as you get into a fierce pose.

- Cross the right elbow over to the left thigh then place your right palm on the mat next to your foot.

- Stretch your left arm towards the ceiling straight as you shift your shoulder and gaze at the lifted palm.

- Ensure that the knees are parallel as you hold in the position for five deep breaths then change to the right side.

Benefits

- Strengthens and stretches the lower legs and aids digestion

- Stimulates the removal of waste from the body.

36. **Shoulder stand pose**

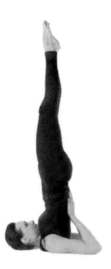

Steps

- Keep your back straight as you raise your legs and your head to the opposite direction.

- You're likely to experience intense pressure on the shoulders.

- Use the palms to support your back and the lower body.

Benefits

- Great exercise for a glowing face. It also relaxes the entire body and toughens the shoulders and upper parts of the body.

37.   **Extended table top**

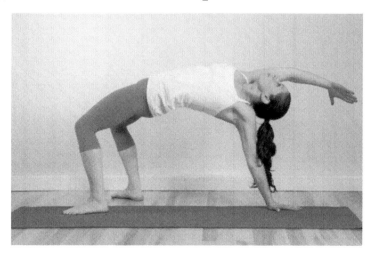

Steps

- Begin by placing both your feet on the mat then lower your left hand on the mat.

- Stretch your right arm straight behind you. Your body should rotate to about 180 degrees as you lift your belly upwards.

- Your feet should be parallel to each other and wide apart

- Hold on to the position as you take five deep breaths then release and repeat the posture about three times.

Benefits

- Enhances flexibility and opens up the front part of the body.

- Stretches and strengthens the muscles and tones the body

- Soothes and stretches the spine, hamstrings, and calves.

- Relieves fatigue and stress

38.   Half Pigeon

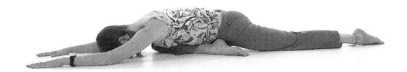

Steps

- Begin by lying on the mat and stretching your right leg forward then bend your right knee and let it overlap until feet touch your left thighs.

- Stretch the right foot straight the on the floor as you also stretch your hands above your head.

- Allow the left leg to rest on the floor as the top of your foot faces down.

- Bring down your head until it touches the mat as shown in the pose.

- Stay in the position as you take five deep breaths then release and repeat with the other leg.

Benefits

- Stimulates the abdominal muscles and the internal organs. It also stretches the deep glutes and helps in toning the body

- Strengthens and stretches the groins.

39. **Killer Praying Mantis**

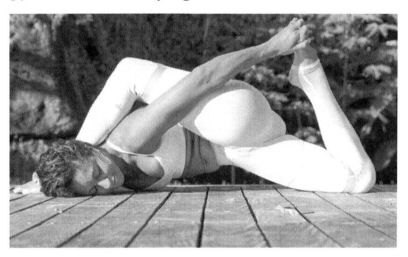

Steps

- Begin by lying on the floor as you also raise your left leg over your head as shown in the pose.

- Fold the right thighs then raise the legs straight as you also stretch the left hand and hold your right feet.

- Bring the left leg close to your neck as your right hands hold on the right leg

- Stay in the posture as you take six deep breaths then relax repeat with the other side.

Benefits

- Strengthens and stretches the muscles in the entire body and also opens up the hips.

- Improves the functioning of the inner organs and increases blood circulation.

40. Cat Pose

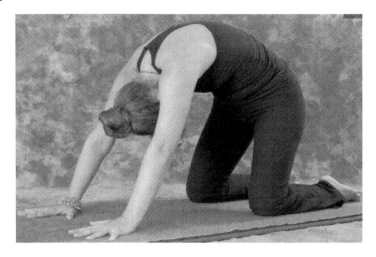

Steps

- Begin with all the four on the mat then bend forward as you raise your hips then place your palms on the mat with your hands and fingers apart.

- Lower your head then raise your torso inwards

- Bring forward your arm then close your knees while you also keep the knees straight.

- Stay in the position as you take ten deep breaths then repeat the pose three times.

Benefits

- Improves body balance and posture

- Stretches and strengthens the abdominal muscles, the spine, and the neck.

- Stretches the hips, the abdomen, and the spine as you also increase coordination.

- Stretches and stimulates belly organs and the abdominal organs

41.Reversed Child's pose

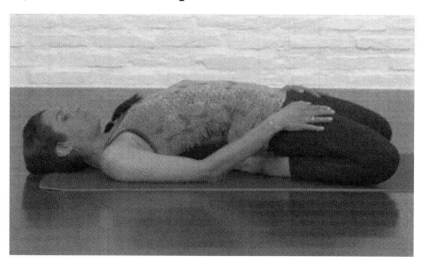

Steps

- Begin by lying on the mat then bend your knees right below the hips as shown in the pose above.

- Lift your hips and allow them to rest on the legs while you place the arms on your thighs

- Lift up your torso while your shoulders and head rest on the floor.

- Stay in the position as you take several deep breaths so as to stay in the position.

Benefits

- Stretches and strengthens the abdominal muscles

- Speeds up digestion and also strengthens the calves and the thigh muscles and the calves

42.   Headstand with lotus legs

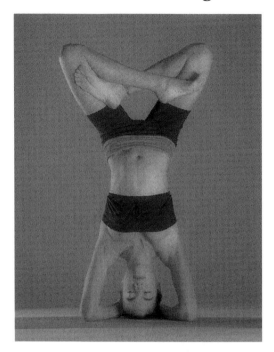

Steps

- Place your head on then with your hands around your head. Then raise one of your legs up as you also try to balance your body.

- Place your arms around your head with your hands held together right behind your head.

- Lift the other leg up then bend and place both the legs together in a lotus pose.

- Stay in the position as you take five deep long breaths.

Benefits

- Improves the flow of blood to the brain and upper body parts and also addresses nervous related issues.

- Improves memory and helps with stress relief.

43.   Arms and a twist

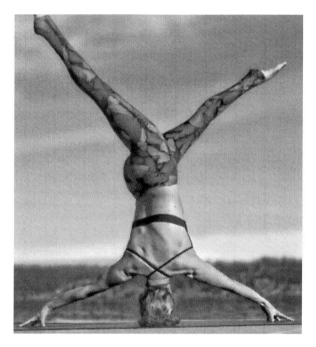

Steps

- Place your head on the mat with your hands wide apart and pressed on the mat.

- Raise one leg upwards as you gain balance then slowly bring the other leg up towards the ceiling.

- Stretch your legs in a twist as shown in the pose above.

- Hold on to the position as you take five deep breaths.

Benefits

- Improves the flow of blood to the brain and also strengthens the upper body muscles.

- Improves body balance and stability.

44.   Crescent Lunge

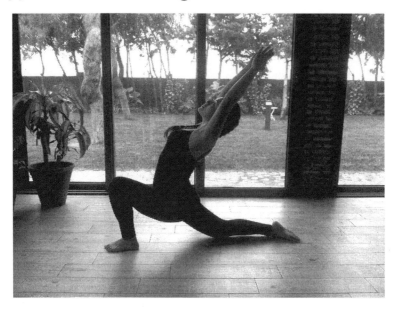

Steps

- Start in a low lunge posture then straighten your back leg with as you also raise your heels.

- Lean backward as you push your torso inwards then stretch both your hands straight up.

- Hold onto the position as you take five deep breaths then turn to the other leg.

Benefits

- Stretches the legs, groins, and the hip flexors

- Strengthens the muscles and tones the hips, thighs, and the butt.

- Enhances flexibility and stability of the body.

45.   Forearm plank

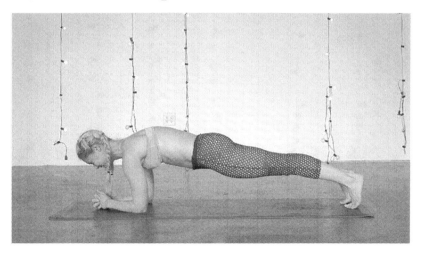

Steps

- Start in a table top position as you place your arms on the mat and the hands held together with fingers pointing forward

- Straighten your legs as you bring them into plank position together with your forearms.

- Push your chest and torso inwards as you also tighten your thighs and butts

- Focus your gaze between your forearms

- Hold on to the position as you take five deep breaths

Benefits

- Improves overall body posture and also tightens the tummy muscles

- Enhances flexibility and overall balance

- Strengthens the core muscles and the spine.

46.   Dolphin pose

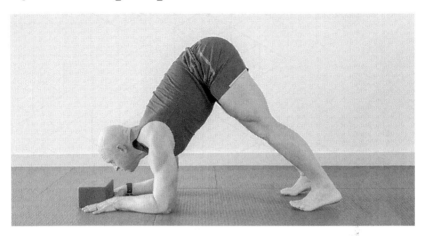

Steps

- Begin by placing both your hands and knees on the mat then stretch your knees beneath the hips.

- Your shoulders should be above the wrists.

- Press your palms on the mat and forearms on the floor.

- Curl your toes as you also lift your knees slightly above the floor then lift your sitting bones upwards

- Firm your shoulder blades against your back while you hold your head raised in between your arms

- Straighten your knees while you also lengthen the tailbone

- Old on to the position and take deep breaths for 30 seconds then release.

Benefits

- Provides relief from fatigue, insomnia, and mild depression
- Provides relief from stress and anxiety
- Improved digestion
- Provides relief from sinusitis, back pain, menstrual discomfort and flat feet and asthma.

47.   Eagle Pose

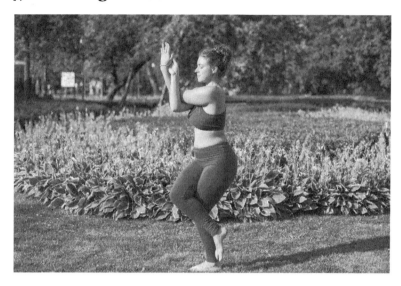

Steps

- Begin in mountain pose with your arms by your sides then bend your knees

- Stretch your arms upwards and twist them in front of your body then bend your elbows as you also raise your forearms so that it's perpendicular to the ground.

- Cross your thighs with your right leg foot placed over the left one.

- Raise your head straight as you gaze at your twisted arms.

- Take several deep breaths then relax and change to the other leg.

Benefits

- Strengthens and stretches the arms, legs, knees, and the joints.

- Strengthens the shoulder blades

48.　　Warrior 11

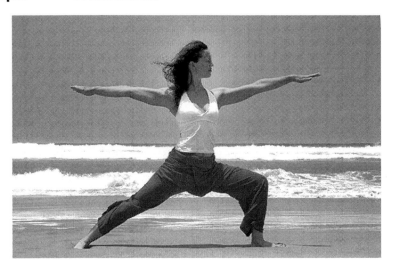

Steps

- Stand straight with your legs apart as you inhale then raise and stretch both of your hands

- Stretch both your legs as you also bend the right knee while keeping your arms and shoulders straight.

- Breathe in as turn towards the front then breathe out as you turn to the right side.

- Repeat the posture several times for about 5 minutes

Benefits

- Strengthens the legs and also opens up the hips and chest

- Improves the level of concentration, focus, balance, and stability

- Improves blood circulation to various parts of the body and energizes the entire body

49.   Headstand bow pose

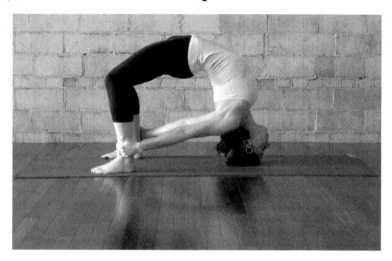

Steps

- Begin by lying on the back then bend your knees as you place your feet flat on the mat and move your heels close

- Bend your elbows then place your palms on the mat right above your shoulders and your fingertips facing your feet

- Lift your head and shoulder from the ground then place your head on the mat.

- Reach out your hand to your feet as you hold onto your ankles

- Stay in that position for about 30 seconds as you take five deep breaths then lower your hips as you let go of your ankles.

Benefits

- Strengthens and stretches your back muscles and also improves the body posture

- Stretches the thighs, ankles, groins, the abdomen, and the chest

- Stimulates abdominal organs

50.   Mermaid in Low Lunge

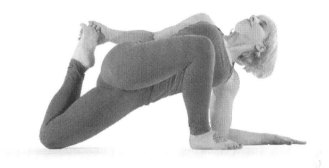

Steps

- Begin in the downward facing dog position then inhale as you also lift your right leg up then step it between your hands.

- Your right ankle will directly be under the knee.

- Lower your back then raise your left knee as you lift your head then rest it on your leg as shown in the pose.

- Lengthen the torso upright then relax your shoulders.

- Stay in the position for about 30 seconds as you hold several breaths then relax and change to the left side.

Benefits

- Cultivates fluidity, and strength.

- Increases strength, flexibility and stability.

- This is the exercise is suitable for those who spend a lot of time in a seated position.

Chapter 5

Guide on Stretching

Engaging in stretching helps in reducing stress, enhances flexibility and re-energizes the body. Engaging in free-range body movement refreshes the body and also enables one to realize their full potential. As a beginner, you should, however ,practice the stretches with caution as there are progressions that may prove to be difficult especially if the muscles are not yet well trained and flexible. It's therefore advisable that you get to know your limits when it comes to yoga stretching. Having some knowledge of stretching techniques that you can use can, however, help with insight on how to go through the process.

Engaging in stretching techniques is important if you intend to realize the following;

- Practice yoga and home and get to improve your flexibility

- Achieve better fitness results from your training by releasing and lengthening tight muscles.

- Get relief from stress as you set your mind to work and meeting busy schedules.

- Improve your yoga practice and get to advanced levels.

- Recover from injury s a result of physical exercise or sport.

- Seek improved joint and muscle functionality with less injury

- Reduce body stiffness and soreness

- Improve in athletic performance for any sport as a beginner or elite.

- Enhance physical exercise regime and weight loss.

An ideal work out and stretching incorporates about six postures and all together helps in improving the alignment of the body, flexibility, strength, and relaxation. Standing poses help in building body strength and stamina. The balancing poses help in improving balance while also promoting focus. The forward bends help in stretching the hamstrings and the back muscles, the back bends and also improves breathing. The twists help in aiding digestion and also tone the abs.

Inversions help in increasing blood circulation which then leaves one feeling energized and calm. The following poses from each of the group including a few modifications can make the practice process much easier for beginners.

Standing forward fold (Standing pose)

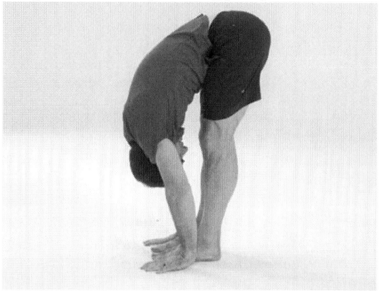

This pose helps in stretching the lower back and hamstrings and its recommended at the beginning of yoga practice. You can engage in the pose as a way of preparation for about 30 seconds then repeat for a maximum of 3 minutes. Remember not to return to standing position fast as you may find yourself feeling dizzy. You can rise up slowly with a strong core.

You can also add modifications to the pose such as a shoulder stretch to the forward fold. You will get to receive the same benefits alongside flexible shoulders.

Downward dog (Inversion pose)

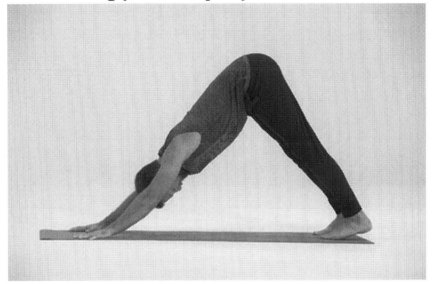

This pose helps in strengthening the arms and the shoulders while also stretching the hamstrings, Achilles tendons and calves. From the wrists to the hips and heels you get to create one straight line. It's advisable that you build up strength as you hold on to the pose for about two minutes. Staying in the pose for 30 seconds may seem to be quite tough for a beginner as you have to bend your knees slightly so as to lengthen your spine. Once you feel exhausted, you can just drop your knees.

Crescent Pose

This pose helps in strengthening and stretching the body at the same time. You get to strengthen the front leg as you also stretch the hip flexor of your back. The pose also improves ability to focus and balance by steadying your gaze in one unmoving point.

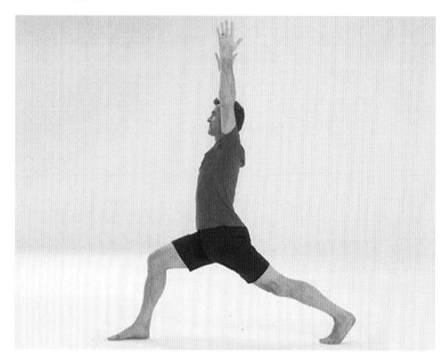

Pyramid pose (back bend pose)

This pose helps in stretching the hamstrings and the lower back. It also strengthens the shin muscles, quadriceps, and feet. Remember to add modifications as desired as you practice the posture.

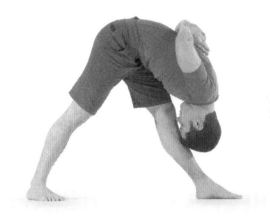

Spinal Twist Pose (Twist pose)

This type of pose is great for increasing the lateral flexibility. It also stretches the spine the shoulders and the neck. Remember not to push too hard when practicing this pose since yoga does not entail feeling pain but relief from pain. In case the back cracks and you don't feel pain then that's fine as it's a sign that the spine is getting realigned. You can modify the twists as desired for enhanced benefits.

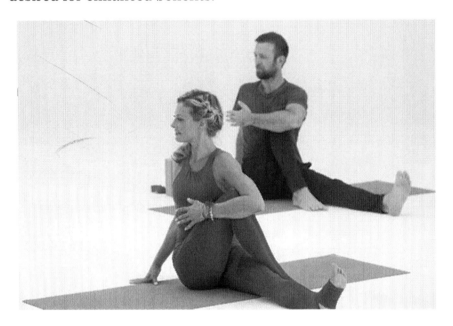

Tree Pose (balance)

This pose helps in improving the overall balance of the body. It also strengthens the core, calves, thighs ankles and the spine. This pose is great when you are working on attaining balance and posture. You can skip engaging in this pose if you have cases of high blood pressure or medical conditions that can affect your balance.

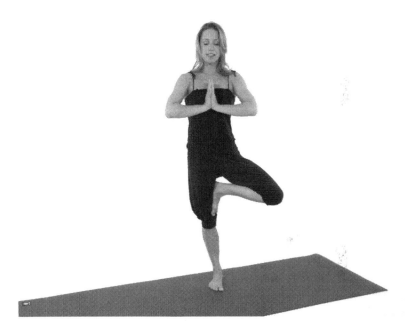

Each of the postures shared above helps in addressing balance, flexibility, stretches and lengthens the muscles and tones the abs. Take your time to practice the stretches you also make appropriate modifications where necessary. Remember that the physical, emotional and mental benefits of yoga are linked. Stretching does not only help with releasing the build-up tension, it also helps with building strength and also boosts self-confidence. Holding onto a pose for just a minute or more can also help in improving focus and improves spiritual insight.

Conclusion

Congratulations and thank you for taking your time to download **Yoga Bible for Beginners**. The book has shared most of the basic and fundamental teachings on yoga and how one can transform their lives and get to live a healthy and fulfilling life by practicing yoga. As a beginner who is just starting out on yoga, it's important that you take time and understand what yoga practice actually entails. It's when you have a clear understanding that you will be able to improve your life and enjoy most of the benefits that come with practicing yoga.

This book has also shared some of the yoga poses that you can begin practicing. Remember that yoga practice is not just about the postures but also entails other steps which the postures prepare you for. To quiet the mind and be able to practice mindfulness and meditation effectively, breathing exercises and postures should be practiced well. As a beginner, start off with postures that you find to be easy and those that your body can easily practice. You don't have to compete with anyone as everyone has a unique path in yoga practice.

Take your time with every step of the practice and remember that it's by practicing consistently that will give you the desired benefits of yoga. If there is an area that you are not clear about then you can go ahead and refer back to the topic for more clarity.

I know you have found the book to be valuable however I have a request; would you please go ahead and leave a review for the book on Amazon.

Thank you and enjoy your new lifestyle!

Printed in Great Britain
by Amazon